Ayan Mondal[1], Atul Kabra*[1]

Advancing Diabetic Wound Healing

Ayan Mondal[1], Atul Kabra*[1]

[1]University Institute of Pharma Sciences,
Chandigarh University, Panjab, India

Correspondence to: Dr. Atul Kabra, Associate
Professor, Chandigarh University, NH05,
Chandigarh-Ludhiana Highway, Gharuan, Mohali,
Punjab -140413, India

1

Ayan Mondal[1], Atul Kabra*[1]

Abstract

Diabetic injuries are exorbitantly prone to infection because of the diabetes damage, suggests delayed and deficient mending ways. Diabetes-related sores and ulcers have led to an increasing medical burden. An abnormal injury Mending is a severe consequence of both type I and type II diabetes and is the most frequent cause of non-traumatic lower branch amputation. Diabetic wound recuperating could be a complex preparation ruined by a few pathophysiological variables, counting microcirculatory unsettling influences and a diminishment in endogenous development variables. Potential wound healing is a dynamic process which includes overlapping phases of haemostasis, inflammation, proliferation, and remodeling. Hyperglycemia, oxidative stress, vascular insufficiency, and microbial infections are all factors that contribute to chronic problems in diabetic patients. Chronic wound healing can be delayed due to infection, excess free radical formation, inflammation, increased protease activity, reduced collagen formation, and decreased production of growth factors like TGF-β, EGF, and VEGF.

Ayan Mondal[1], Atul Kabra*[1]

Throughout the research it helps to understand that specifically targeted treatment requires diabetic foot ulcers. For the early and effective intervention and wound management strategies are various type of drug delivery – including nanoparticles hydrogels, dendrimers, liposomes, with incorporated bioactive agents and biological macromolecules also use. This review highlights the potential of novel approaches such as anti-microbials, minerals, vitamins, development variables quality treatment, and stem cell-based treatment in diabetic wound mending. However, the translation from research to clinical application remains challenging and concerted efforts are needed to bridge this gap. As the field continues to evolve, integrating innovative therapies into existing treatment protocols offers has potential to significantly improve the outcomes for individuals with diabetes.

Future research should focus on overcoming barriers to clinical application so that knowledge gained from clinical research can be effectively applied in real-world settings to improve wound healing in patients with diabetes.

Keywords: Diabetes mellitus; Foot ulceration; Ulcer treatment strategies; wound healing

Ayan Mondal[1], Atul Kabra*[1]

Table of content

Ayan Mondal[1], Atul Kabra*[1]

Introduction

Diabetic foot ulcers (DFUs) are a frequent and dangerous consequence of diabetes. It is predicted that 15% to 25% of people with diabetes will acquire DFU throughout their lives. Globally, this results in millions of people being affected. Currently, around 463 million people worldwide are living with diabetes, according to the International Diabetes Federation (IDF, 2019), the number of people affected is projected to be 600 million by 2035. The most prevalent types of diabetes are type 1 diabetes mellitus (T1DM) and type 2 diabetes mellitus (T2DM) with both strong heritable components. In addition, there are other specific causes of diabetes, including: diabetes of young adults and diabetes caused by mitochondrial gene mutations. Diabetic wound healing is frequently delayed due to underlying ischemia, infection, neuropathic, and metabolic problems. Diabetic wounds are a type of persistent, refractory ulcer. It is often caused by microcirculatory abnormalities, low levels of endogenous growth factors. Diabetic foot ulcer (DFU) is a common and deadly consequence of diabetes mellitus, characterized by the development of lower extremity ulcers and gangrene caused by macro- and microvascular lesions.

Ayan Mondal[1], Atul Kabra*[1]

One of the common chronic complications of diabetes is the delayed cutaneous wound healing. The cutaneous wound healing process in diabetics is affected by various interrelated factors including hyperglycemia, excess free radical production, oxidative stress, vascular insufficiency, microbial infections, excessive inflammation, and even increased protease action, among others. Any of the following processes may contribute to the observed tendency: an increase in the number of growth factor cells such as TGF-β, EGF and VEGF. The objectives outlined in this article will help come up with the reasons as to why the wound healing is uncommon in diabetic patients and will outline various research papers that aim to explain the peculiarities in the patients.

Wound healing cannot occur in the absence of macrophages. During wound healing, invading macrophages deployed at the inflammatory phase are described as the M1 phenotype as they fight off invading bacteria and necrotic tissue. They subsequently change into anti-inflammatory macrophages of the M2 phenotype, therefore enhancing the processes of regeneration phase of wound healing. Impaired macrophage polarization toward the M2 phenotype results in a prolonged "mild inflammatory phase" in diabetic wounds.

Several materials have been developed to treat DFUs, some of which have been authorized by the US FDA. For example, Acellular Dermal Matrix, an

Ayan Mondal[1], Atul Kabra*[1]

extracellular matrix-based material, permits cell infiltration and proliferation, which promotes vascularization, matrix deposition, and re-epithelialization. The Integra Dermal Regeneration Template, a product of Integra Life Sciences in the United States, is one example with FDA approval.

Although various treatments for diabetic wound healing have been developed in recent years, diabetic ulcers remain a significant clinical challenge. Furthermore, the goal is to investigate treatment strategies that target these pathways, such as increasing growth factor production. The ultimate goal is to create successful ways for expediting wound healing in diabetic patients and increasing their quality of life.

Ayan Mondal[1], Atul Kabra*[1]

Diabetic Wounds and Diabetic Foot Ulcers

A wound is described as a break in the skin, mucous membrane, or tissue. Wounds can also be classified as acute (healing within 3 weeks) or chronic (taking 6 weeks to heal).

The principles of wound healing

Wound healing is an ongoing and complicated procedure that starts when tissue integrity is compromised. Healing is split into four overlapping phases: hemostatic, inflammatory, proliferative, and remodeling.

Hemostasis

Platelets serve an important part in hemostasis, the initial process in tissue rebuild. When circulation platelets are exposed to collagen in injured cells, they activate, aggregate, and attach to the injured epithelium.

Activation of the process of coagulation results in conversion of fibrinogen to fibrin, resulting in a clot and a reserve extracellular matrix.

Platelets were released proteins that stimulate neutrophil, monocyte migration and adhesion, as well as growth factors including platelet-derived

8

Ayan Mondal[1], Atul Kabra*[1]

growth factor (PDGF) and transforming growth factor b (TGF-b), which promote wound healing.

Inflammation Phase

The incendiary stage of wound healing begins shortly after damage, when incendiary cells attack the injury.

Neutrophils are the first cells to enter injured tissue. Adhesion molecules on the vascular endothelial surface near the injured tissue become activated, causing neutrophils to adhere to the endothelium. The neutrophils then migrate deeper into the tissue space via ruptured capillaries or between endothelial cells (dialysis). Neutrophils help to manage infections and debride tissues.

They also contribute to wound healing by producing growth factors that stimulate cell proliferation and proteases that break down the extracellular matrix. Circulating monocytes penetrate the tissue area and quickly develop into adult macrophages, causing inflammation.

Active or pro-inflammatory macrophages (M1 macrophages) remove pathogens, foreign substances, dying neutrophils, and damaged tissue elements from the site of injury by phagocytosis. They also generate many pro-inflammatory mediators, including cytokines. Resident mast cells react fast to injury to tissue and play a key role in the wound recovery process.

Ayan Mondal[1], Atul Kabra*[1]

Mast cells degranulate, producing cytokines that promote neutrophil recruitment and protein enzymes that break down the matrix of cells. T cells infiltrate the location during the late inflammatory phase and may influence remodeling of tissue.

Proliferative Phase

The injury undergoes a proliferative phase as inflammation subsides and macrophages switch to an alternative activation or anti-inflammatory phenotype.

Anti-inflammatory macrophages (M2 macrophages) produce a variety of anti-inflammatory mediators, proteases, and protease inhibitors, as well as growth factors such as VEGF, EGF, FGF, IL8, and TGF-b, which promote cell proliferation and protein synthesis.

Granulation tissue begins to replace the temporary matrix in the wound.

Growth factors generated by macrophages activate fibroblasts, which migrate into the wound and use the temporary matrix as a scaffold.

Here, they begin, multiply and make collagen and other extracellular matrix components.

The development of new capillaries promotes the proliferation of fibroblast growth factors. New blood capillaries must be formed from pre-existing

Ayan Mondal[1], Atul Kabra*[1]

capillary networks in order to provide oxygen and nutrients to the wound's rapidly expanding cells.

Angiogenesis, on the other hand, involves the formation of new blood vessels by recruiting progenitor cells (endothelial progenitor cells, or EPCs) from the bone marrow. EPCs are an adult stem cell population that can differentiate into epithelial cells and promote endothelium regeneration and angiogenesis in response to tissue hypoxia.

Angiogenesis is a dynamic and carefully regulated process that depends primarily on pro-angiogenic hormones, such as FGF-2 and VEGF, and anti-angiogenic factors acting on endothelial cells.

FGF-2 appears to be released secondary to tissue damage during the first three days of wound healing, whereas VEGF release after the first three days is predominantly triggered by tissue hypoxia.

During the early phases of proliferation, new capillaries establish a microvascular network across the granulation tissue. Blood artery density diminishes as the healing process progresses.

Granulation tissue is a new connective tissue distinguished by its characteristic granular appearance induced by the presence of numerous new capillaries.

It is formed during the healing process and is made up of fibroblasts, endothelial cells, inflammatory

11

Ayan Mondal[1], Atul Kabra*[1]

cells, extracellular matrix components, and new blood vessels. Keratinocytes move from the wound edges or adjacent skin appendages onto the new matrix, causing re-epithelialization, which covers the granulation tissue and bridges the wound.

The wounded epidermis releases several growth factors, including endothelial growth factor (EGF), keratinocyte growth factor, and FGF-2, which encourage epithelial proliferation.

Remodeling Phase

The fourth cycle of wound treatment, known as remodeling, is considered the most clinically relevant. The reconstitution stage of healing a wound occurs roughly 2-3 weeks after the initial injury, when granulation adipose tissue gradually converts into mature scar tissue. This stage aims to reach grain maturity and maximum tensile strength by rebuilding, disintegrating, and renewing the extracellular matrix (ECM).

The newly manufactured the fibers of collagen are no more haphazardly positioned, but are more precisely spaced along stress lines, promoting cross-linking and thereby increasing the wound's tensile strength. This process is regulated by many growth factors, including TGF-1 and FGF, as well as cytokines like IL-10, which inhibit chemokine synthesis.

Ayan Mondal[1], Atul Kabra*[1]

Wound contraction also occurs, with myofibroblasts pulling the wound edges towards each other, thereby reducing the size of the wound.

Ayan Mondal[1], Atul Kabra*[1]

Wound phase	Characteristics in diabetic wounds
Haemostasis	A procoagulant state usually occurs, in which fibrinolysis is impaired, causing occlusion of small capillaries.
Inflammation	These wounds are halted during the inflammatory stage. The intense infiltration of neutrophils and monocytes becomes persistent. Inflammatory cells avoid apoptosis, disrupting the wound healing process. Local cytokine secretion inhibits the transcription of growth factor genes for extracellular matrix production and angiogenesis.
Granulation tissue	The chemotaxis of

Ayan Mondal[1], Atul Kabra*[1]

formation	fibroblasts and fibrocytes to the wound has diminished. Fibroblast and endothelial cell multiplication are slowed or stopped, and apoptosis is common. Extracellular matrix secretion is reduced, resulting in reduced tensile strength and poorer cell anchoring. Myofibroblast differentiation has reduced. Alpha-smooth muscle synthesis is inhibited, resulting in extremely restricted wound contraction. Angiogenic responses are compromised, resulting in tissue perfusion abnormalities. Hyperglycemia inhibits angiogenesis and endothelial nitric oxide production. The control of

Ayan Mondal[1], Atul Kabra*[1]

	microcapillary tone is disturbed.
Re-epithelialization	Epithelial pre-migration and proper keratinocyte implicit differentiation are compromised, resulting in delayed wound healing. Re-epithelialization is slow and may not be successful for months or years.
Remodeling	Removal of the bluff matrix and replacement with a more typical active matrix happens gradually, increasing the danger of re-ulceration.

Ayan Mondal[1], Atul Kabra*[1]

1.Microcirculatory disturbances and reduced endogenous growth factors

In diabetes, excessive blood sugar levels can damage small blood vessels, resulting in impaired circulation and oxygen delivery to tissues. This disorder, called microangiopathy, impairs the body's capacity to heal wounds properly.

The most frequent diabetes complications are retinopathy, neuropathy, nephropathy, peripheral vascular disease, and diabetic foot syndrome. Microcirculation is a key factor in all of these issues.

In patients with diabetes, there is a notable presence of endothelial damage and microvascular dysfunction in various regions of the body, such as the eyes, kidneys, and feet. Microvascular damage, both structural and functional (referred to as microangiopathy or small vessel disease), is frequently seen in diabetic individuals due to glycation-related alterations stemming from a sustained hyperglycemic condition. The significance of microcirculation in diabetic foot ulcers is a subject of ongoing investigation, with numerous studies on microcirculation presenting various theories, including the idea of "small vessel disease." Research has also indicated that arteriovenous shunting resulting from sympathetic

17

Ayan Mondal[1], Atul Kabra*[1]

denervation elevates capillary pressure in the feet of individuals with diabetes.

Ayan Mondal[1], Atul Kabra*[1]

Reduced Placenta Growth Factor (PlGF):

Diabetic wounds exhibit diminished expression of PlGF, which hinders angiogenesis, a crucial process for effective wound healing. In diabetic wounds, the downregulation of growth factor alpha-receptor coupled with the swift degradation of growth factors results in a prolonged healing process. Among these vital growth factors is pDGF, a serum mitogen released by platelets that significantly facilitates fibroblast proliferation, matrix organization, and the development of connective tissue. During the late inflammatory phase, macrophages generate pDGF within the wound environment, attracting fibroblasts and inflammatory cells due to its pro-proliferative attributes. This combination subsequently a

Abstract

Introduction

Diabetic Wounds and Diabetic Foot Ulcers

2. Pathophysiology Associated with Diabetic Wound Healing

4. Conventional Wound Care Techniques

8.Conclusion

ids in the synthesis of collagen, glycosaminoglycans, proteoglycans, and glycans, culminating in the creation of granulation tissue proteins, a provisional extracellular matrix, and

19

Ayan Mondal[1], Atul Kabra*[1]

angiogenesis. The overexpression of PlGF or the implementation of gene therapy to introduce PlGF notably hastens wound healing by fostering tissue formation and angiogenesis.

Vascular Endothelial Growth Factor (VEGF):

VEGF is a potent angiogenic cytokine abundantly found in the skin, and its concentration within wounds is pivotal to the healing process. Through vasculogenesis and angiogenesis, it supports the critical phases while promoting the proteolytic degradation of blood vessels located within the extracellular matrix. VEGF elicits migration and proliferation of endothelial cells. In general, VEGF stimulates capillary densities; together, these actions augment blood flow and metabolic, promote granulation tissue formation, with an impact on wound protein levels, which contribute to the regulation of re-vascularization and permeability levels. This factor acts through receptors; the VEGF receptors 1 and 2 nature are very critical to starting inflammation and angiogenesis. In the diabetic state, reduced expression of VEGF causes a reduction in angiogenesis. Therapies seeking to restore VEGF action may be able to revive this activity and thus further promote angiogenesis and wound healing.

Basic Fibroblast Growth Factor (FGF-2):

BFGF is involved in several biological processes, like fibroblast growth and differentiation,

Ayan Mondal[1], Atul Kabra*[1]

stimulation of vascular smooth muscle and endothelial cells, extracellular matrix metabolism, and migration of mesodermal cells. In this way, it induces the formation of granulation tissue, accelerating the healing process by stimulating the functions of the cells concerned.

bFGF could enhance both the rate and the extent of granulation tissue formation, significantly influencing the wound healing process.

In the diabetic environment, glycation downregulates the activity of FGF-2, affecting capillary formation and giving rise to poor wound healing. Glycation compromises the ability of FGF-2 to bind to its receptor, thus undermining its healing potential.

Keratinocyte Growth Factor (KGF):

In diabetic wounds, reduced and inhibited KGF expression inhibits re-epithelialization, which is required for the healing process.

Growth factor family

The family of growth factors is crucial in the process of wound healing, with a variety of growth factors derived from different cellular origins that perform a range of biological functions. Fibroblast growth factors (FGFs), which include acidic FGF, basic FGF, and keratinocyte growth factor (KGF), are synthesized by macrophages, endothelial cells, and fibroblasts, promoting angiogenesis, the

Ayan Mondal[1], Atul Kabra*[1]

activation of endothelial cells, as well as the proliferation and migration of keratinocytes, and the deposition of extracellular matrix (ECM) (Huang, S.M. et al., 2019). Transforming growth factors (TGF-β), such as TGF-β1, TGF-β2, and TGF-β3, derived from platelets, fibroblasts, and macrophages, enhance fibroblast chemotaxis and activation, ECM deposition, collagen production, and the generation of tissue inhibitors of metalloproteinases (TIMPs) and matrix metalloproteinases (MMPs), while also minimizing scarring (Fanxing Xu et al., 2013). Platelet-derived growth factors (PDGFs), which consist of PDGF-AA, PDGF-BB, and vascular endothelial growth factors (VEGF), are secreted by platelets, macrophages, keratinocytes, and fibroblasts; they stimulate immune and fibroblast cells, assist in ECM deposition, and encourage angiogenesis (Bizunesh M. Borena et al., 2015). Connective tissue growth factor (CTGF), which is secreted by fibroblasts, endothelial cells, and epithelial cells, regulates the effects of TGF-β on collagen production (Richard W.D. Gilbert et al., 2016). Furthermore, insulin-like growth factors (IGFs), including IGF-I and IGF-II, produced by the liver, skeletal muscle, fibroblasts, macrophages, and neutrophils, facilitate keratinocyte proliferation, the activation of endothelial cells, fibroblast proliferation, angiogenesis, collagen production, and overall cellular metabolism (Ming O. Li et al., 2006). Finally, epidermal growth factors (EGFs),

Ayan Mondal[1], Atul Kabra*[1]

such as EGF, HB-EGF, TGF-β, amphiregulin, and betacellulin, primarily sourced from keratinocytes and macrophages, stimulate keratinocyte proliferation and migration, as well as ECM deposition (Shentong Fang et al., 2012). Collectively, these growth factors synchronize the intricate processes essential for successful wound healing and tissue restoration.

Cytokines involved in wound healing

Anti-inflammatory and pro-inflammatory cytokines are critical in wound healing because they influence many cellular activities. T-cells, macrophages, and keratinocytes secrete anti-inflammatory cytokines such as IL-10, which inhibit the synthesis of pro-inflammatory cytokines such as TNF, IL-1, and IL-6 while also dampening the activation of macrophages and polymorphonuclear leukocytes (PMNs) (Riichiro Abe et al., 2001). Similarly, T-cells, basophils, and mast cells release IL-4, which suppresses TNF, IL-1, and IL-6 production, boosting fibroblast proliferation and collagen creation (Boris Hinz et al., 2007). Pro-inflammatory cytokines like as IL-8, which are produced by PMNs, fibroblasts, and macrophages, improve macrophage and PMN chemotaxis while also assisting keratinocyte maturation (J.M. Reinke et al., 2012). Macrophages produce IL-1, which increases collagen synthesis and fibroblast and keratinocyte chemotaxis (Boris Hinz et al., 2003). IL-2, a keratinocyte and T-cell-produced cytokine,

23

Ayan Mondal[1], Atul Kabra*[1]

increases fibroblast infiltration and activity. Macrophages produce IL-6, which promotes fibroblast proliferation and hepatic acute-phase protein synthesis (Berlanga-Acosta et al., 2020). Fibroblasts and T-cells produce γ-Interferon, which activates macrophages and PMNs but may inhibit collagen synthesis and cross-linking (Sohini Sen et al., 2020). TNF-β, released by macrophages, promotes PMN margination, cytotoxicity, collagen formation, and metabolic substrates (Kaihua Zhang et al., 2001). These cytokines work together to coordinate the complex mechanisms required for proper wound healing.

Ayan Mondal[1], Atul Kabra*[1]

2. Pathophysiology Associated with Diabetic Wound Healing

Diabetic sores, particularly foot ulcers, are a major consequence of diabetes and significantly contribute to the illness's morbidity. These wounds do not heal properly because to a range of variables that disrupt the usual wound healing process, including poor angiogenesis, chronic inflammation, neuropathy, and a reduced immunological response. Understanding these fundamental principles is critical for developing effective methods to improve wound healing in people with diabetes.

Impaired Angiogenesis in Diabetes

Angiogenesis, or the process by which new blood vessels form from old ones, is essential for tissue repair and wound healing. This process is significantly slowed in those with diabetes. Elevated blood sugar levels cause endothelial cell dysfunction, which is required for the development of new blood vessels. Diabetic conditions reduce the synthesis of vascular endothelial growth factor (VEGF), a key component in angiogenesis. As a result, the decreased creation of blood vessels reduces the flow of oxygen and critical nutrients to the wound region, slowing the healing process.

Additionally, elevated glucose levels lead to the creation of advanced glycation end-products (AGEs), which further disrupt angiogenesis. AGEs

25

Ayan Mondal[1], Atul Kabra*[1]

attach their receptors on various cells, including endothelial cells, resulting in oxidative stress and inflammation. These alterations interfere with the normal signaling necessary for the proliferation and migration of endothelial cells, worsening the already compromised wound healing situation in diabetic individuals.

Chronic Inflammation in Diabetic Wounds

While inflammation is a typical and vital aspect of wound healing, in the case of diabetic wounds, this phase often becomes extended and chronic. The elevated blood glucose levels foster a pro-inflammatory environment that hinders the shift from the inflammatory phase to the proliferative phase of healing. Chronic inflammation is characterized by the ongoing recruitment of immune cells such as neutrophils and macrophages to the wound site. These cells generate an excess of inflammatory cytokines, including tumor necrosis factor-alpha (TNF-α) and interleukins, which prolong tissue damage and obstruct the healing process.

In diabetes, the dysregulation of these inflammatory pathways also results in a delayed transition of macrophages from the pro-inflammatory M1 phenotype to the anti-inflammatory M2 phenotype. The ongoing presence of M1 macrophages leads to continuous tissue damage and prevents the resolution of inflammation, ultimately hindering wound closure.

Ayan Mondal[1], Atul Kabra*[1]

Neuropathy and Its Role in Wound Formation

Diabetic neuropathy, a widespread complication of diabetes, plays a crucial role in the formation of diabetic wounds, particularly foot ulcers. Neuropathy arises from prolonged hyperglycemia, which harms peripheral nerves and results in a loss of sensation, especially in the lower limbs. Patients suffering from diabetic neuropathy may remain oblivious to minor injuries or pressure points on their feet, allowing these unnoticed wounds to evolve into chronic ulcers.

Moreover, the absence of sensation results in abnormal pressure distribution during walking, leading to repetitive trauma to specific areas of the foot. This ongoing, unrecognized damage culminates in the development of ulcers, which heal slowly due to other diabetic complications such as inadequate blood flow and chronic inflammation.

Impaired Immune Response in Diabetic Patients

Diabetes also reduces the immune system's ability to respond appropriately to wounds. Hyperglycemia impacts various immune system components, including neutrophil function, macrophage activity, and total infection clearance. Neutrophils, which are among the first to respond to a wound, show impaired chemotaxis and phagocytic capacity in diabetic individuals. This limits their ability to combat infections and remove dead tissue from the wound site.

27

Ayan Mondal[1], Atul Kabra*[1]

Macrophages, which play an important role in wound healing by phagocytizing debris and supporting tissue repair, are similarly impaired in diabetes. As previously stated, the failure to transition from the M1 to M2 phenotype impedes inflammation resolution and slows healing. Furthermore, reduced production of cytokines and growth factors by immune cells decreases the body's ability to efficiently repair tissue.

Ayan Mondal[1], Atul Kabra*[1]

3. Challenges in Diabetic Wound Healing

Wound healing in people with diabetes presents major clinical challenges due to the interaction of multiple physiological factors. Diabetics are more prone to wound complications, largely due to hyperglycaemia, poor circulation, increased infection risk, and the frequent occurrence of foot ulcers, which can lead to amputations.

Hyperglycemia and Delayed Wound Healing

Impact of Hyperglycaemia on Wound Healing High blood sugar (hyperglycaemia) disrupts several stages of the wound healing process, prolonging inflammation, impairing white blood cell function, and reducing collagen production, all which delay healing. The weakened immune system also increases the chance of infection.

Infection Risk in Diabetic Wounds Due to both hyperglycaemia and immune system impairment, diabetic wounds are highly prone to infection. Poor circulation and diminished immune response allow bacteria to thrive, complicating healing and potentially leading to severe outcomes like sepsis.

Poor Circulation and Peripheral Artery Disease (PAD) Many people with diabetes also suffer from poor blood circulation, often caused by peripheral artery disease (PAD). PAD reduces blood flow to the extremities, particularly the legs and feet,

Ayan Mondal[1], Atul Kabra*[1]

limiting the supply of oxygen and nutrients to wounds, which delays healing and raises the risk of chronic wounds.

Foot Ulcers and Amputations

A Common Diabetic Complication Foot ulcers are a common and serious complication in diabetics, often resulting from neuropathy (loss of foot sensation), poor circulation, and delayed healing. If not properly treated, foot ulcers can lead to gangrene and, in many cases, the need for amputation. Diabetes is one of the leading causes of non-traumatic lower-limb amputations globally

Ayan Mondal[1], Atul Kabra*[1]

4. Conventional Wound Care Techniques

Debridement is the process of removing necrotic (dead) tissue, debris, or infected tissue from a wound in order to aid healing. Debridement can be carried out surgically, enzymatically, or by autolytic mechanisms. Removing dead tissue reduces bacterial load and provides an ideal environment for new tissue growth.

Dressings: Wound dressings differ according to the nature and severity of the wound. Conventional dressings include:

Hydrocolloids promote autolytic debridement by keeping the wound wet.

Foam dressings absorb exudates while also providing cushioning to protect the wound.

Alginate Dressings: Made from seaweed, these are used to keep moisture balanced in severely exudative wounds.

Antimicrobial Dressings: These dressings, which contain silver or iodine, serve to prevent or treat infections.

Antibiotics and Antimicrobial Agents

Ayan Mondal[1], Atul Kabra*[1]

Diabetic wounds, particularly when infected, necessitate the use of antibiotics to reduce bacterial development. Systemic antibiotics are commonly used to treat infected wounds, whereas topical antimicrobial medicines (such as silver sulfadiazine or iodine) are given directly to the wound.

Antibiotics could be:

Topical: Apply directly to the wound to treat localized infections.

Systemic: Used orally or intravenously to treat deep or widespread illnesses.

Negative pressure wound therapy (NPWT)

Negative Pressure Wound Therapy (NPWT), also known as vacuum-assisted closure, is a sophisticated procedure that employs a vacuum to aid wound healing. A specific dressing is placed to the wound and sealed with an airtight bandage. A suction pump generates negative pressure on the wound, which helps:

- Remove exudates and infectious materials.
- Promote tissue granulation.
- Increase blood flow to the wounded area.

Mechanism:

The negative pressure draws the wound edges together, hastens the production of granulation tissue, and encourages the creation of healthy tissue.

Ayan Mondal[1], Atul Kabra[*1]

The suction also helps to reduce bacterial burden and keep the environment wet, which promotes healing.

Hyperbaric oxygen therapy (HBOT)

Hyperbaric Oxygen Therapy (HBOT) is another sophisticated treatment option for improving oxygen delivery to diabetic wounds. In this therapy, patients are placed in a pressurized chamber and breathe 100% oxygen. Pressurized oxygen allows:

Increased oxygen levels in the blood and tissues enhance cellular repair and speed up the wound healing process.

Improved immunity and angiogenesis (the development of new blood vessels).

The risk of infection is reduced by preventing the growth of anaerobic bacteria.

HBOT is very useful for non-healing ulcers and wounds with significant tissue hypoxia.

The complex nature of diabetic wounds, specifically foot ulcers, needs the development of innovative technologies and medicines that address the underlying pathophysiological issues.

5.Emerging Technologies and Therapies for Diabetic Wound Healing

Traditional therapies, such as wound dressings and antibiotics, frequently fail to speed up healing in

Ayan Mondal[1], Atul Kabra*[1]

severe or chronic wounds. New treatments, such as development factor-based therapies, stem cell therapy, platelet-rich plasma (PRP) therapy, and biomaterials for skin regeneration, provide diabetic patients new hope. These treatments attempt to stimulate tissue repair, boost angiogenesis, and reduce inflammation by targeting the cellular and molecular mechanisms that cause poor wound healing.

Growth Factor-Based Therapies

Growth factors are naturally occurring proteins that influence cellular processes such as growth, division, and migration, all of which play critical roles in wound healing. Diabetic wounds usually show insufficient expression of these growth factors, resulting in poor healing. Growth factor-based therapies aim to address this imbalance by administering exogenous growth factors directly to the wound site.

Vascular endothelial growth factor (VEGF) is a well-studied growth factor that stimulates angiogenesis, the formation of new blood vessels. The topical use of VEGF or similar substances, such as platelet-derived growth factor (PDGF), has shown promise in promoting blood vessel formation, improving oxygen and nutrient delivery to the wound, and enhancing tissue repair. Clinical studies have revealed that recombinant PDGF promotes wound closure in diabetic ulcers.

Ayan Mondal[1], Atul Kabra*[1]

Stem Cell Therapy and Tissue Engineering

Stem cell therapy is an attractive treatment option for diabetic wounds since it has the ability to repair damaged tissues using the body's natural healing mechanisms. Stem cells, particularly those derived from mesenchymal stem cells (MSCs), can differentiate into a range of cell types, including fibroblasts, keratinocytes, and endothelial cells, which are required for wound healing. MSCs also create bioactive compounds that promote angiogenesis, decrease inflammation, and aid in tissue healing. These cells not only actively contribute to tissue regeneration, but they also create an environment that promotes the activity of other cells involved in the healing process. In addition to MSCs, induced pluripotent stem cells (iPSCs) and embryonic stem cells (ESCs) are being investigated for restorative potential, but ethical and safety concerns must be addressed before widespread adoption.

Platelet-Rich Plasma (PRP) Therapy

Platelet-rich plasma (PRP) therapy is a new treatment for diabetic wounds that utilizes platelets, a kind of blood cell responsible for clotting and tissue repair. PRP is made by centrifuging a person's blood to concentrate platelets, which are then applied to a wound. Platelets release growth factors (VEGF, PDGF, and TGF-β) that promote cell proliferation, collagen synthesis, and angiogenesis.

Ayan Mondal[1], Atul Kabra*[1]

Biomaterials and Scaffolds for Skin Regeneration

Biomaterials and scaffolds are an important area of innovation in wound healing because they provide structural support for tissue regeneration while simultaneously acting as delivery vehicles for cells, growth hormones, and medications. These materials are designed to mimic the extracellular matrix (ECM), creating a scaffolding for new tissue formation while also encouraging cell mobility, development, and differentiation.

Natural biomaterials including collagen, hyaluronic acid, and chitosan are commonly employed in healing wounds due to their bio compatibility and ability to stimulate tissue repair. Synthetic polymers, such as polylactic acid (PLA) and polyglycolic acid (PGA), are being investigated for their tenable characteristics and controlled degradation rates. Hybrid materials, which blend natural and synthetic components, provide advantages of both, resulting in scaffolds that are both physiologically active and mechanically strong.

PRP therapy has grown in popularity due to its ease of planning, low risk of rejection (because it uses the patient's own blood), and ability to activate several components of the healing process for wounds.

Ayan Mondal[1], Atul Kabra*[1]

6. Improvements in wound care and delivery systems

Recent advances in wound care have resulted in new dressings and drug delivery systems that not only protect wounds, but also actively encourage healing and infection prevention. Smart dressings with controlled drug release, bioactive compounds, and nanotechnology-based solutions that improve wound treatment outcomes are examples of innovative technologies.

Smart Healing Dressing for Controlled Drug Release

Smart wound dressings are a significant advancement in wound care. These dressings are designed to release therapeutic medications in a controlled and sustained manner in response to environmental stimuli like temperature, pH, and moisture levels in the wound. This allows for a more precise and efficient drug delivery system that responds to the wound's healing requirements.

Smart dressings usually include polymers or hydrogels that encapsulate the medicament. These materials can be programmed to respond to certain triggers, such as a rise in wound pH (a sign of infection), by releasing antibacterial medications, growth hormones, or other drugs.

Ayan Mondal[1], Atul Kabra*[1]

Bioactive Compounds in Dressings

Biological activity bandages have gained popularity due to their ability to interact with injury environments and aid in healing through biological processes. These types of dressings include naturally derived bioactive compounds that enhance wound healing, reduce inflammation, and protect against infection.

Honey-Based Dressings

Honey, particularly honey from Manuka trees, has been traditionally used in wound treatment for its antimicrobial, anti-inflammatory, and wound-healing properties. Honey generates a moist wound environment, encourages the removal of autolytic debris, and its high sugar content prevents bacterial growth via osmosis.

Chitosan-Based Dressings: Chitosan, derived from chitosan (found in shellfish), is a bioactive molecule that aids wound healing by promoting hemostasis, antibacterial activity, and tissue repair. Chitosan dressings are commonly used in trauma and surgical injuries due to its rapid healing qualities.

Ayan Mondal[1], Atul Kabra*[1]

Nanotechnology-Based Wound Dressings

Nanotechnology has transformed wound care by providing more accurate and efficient delivery systems, accelerating healing, and reducing infections. Nanoparticles can be included into wound dressings to transport antibacterial medicines, growth factors, or other therapeutic compounds directly to the wound site on a nanoscale, improving the dressing's interaction with the wound environment.

Nanofibers and Nanoparticles: Nanofiber dressings, usually made of polymers like polyurethane or chitosan, have a highly porous structure that mimics the extracellular matrix, facilitating cell proliferation and tissue regeneration. Nanoparticles, including silver or gold nanoparticles, may be embedded in nanofibers to provide a long-lasting antibacterial effect.

7.Future Directions in Diabetic Wound Care

Technological innovations and personalized therapy are transforming diabetic wound care. Significant focus areas include the incorporation of artificial intelligence (AI), personalized treatment procedures, and the ongoing research of novel medicines. These developments aim to improve healing outcomes and reduce problems.

Ayan Mondal[1], Atul Kabra*[1]

AI plays a critical role in the management of diabetic wounds. Machine learning and computer vision can successfully evaluate wound characteristics such as size, depth, and infection status, providing real-time information to guide treatment decisions. AI-powered systems also track wound growth, forecast healing outcomes, and allow for remote monitoring via telemedicine platforms, which is especially beneficial to patients in underserved areas.

Personalized medicine tailors' therapies to individual genetic, environmental, and behavioral variables. Genomic analysis helps healthcare providers uncover indicators that influence wound healing, paving the way for more targeted treatments. Pharmacogenomics can further customize treatment regimens depending on a patient's drug metabolism, increasing efficacy while reducing side effects. To develop comprehensive solutions, tailored care plans take into account comorbid illnesses such as obesity or cardiovascular difficulties.

Current research and clinical investigations are looking into new remedies, such as gene therapy and nanotechnology-based treatments. Gene therapy aims to improve healing of wounds by increasing the creation of growth factors such as VEGF, which promotes angiogenesis. Nanotechnology enables targeted administration of drugs and growth factors, as well as the development of advanced wound

Ayan Mondal[1], Atul Kabra*[1]

dressings. The development of bioengineered tissue grafts and skin substitutes is also undertaken to improve skin regeneration in chronic wounds. Furthermore, systemic treatments aiming at addressing chronic inflammation and immunological dysfunction are being investigated in order to boost the body's natural healing response. These advancements represent the future of better diabetes wound treatment.

8.Conclusion

Diabetic wound care is embarking on an exciting journey of innovation and change, fueled by technological advances and a deeper understanding of customized therapy. The increasing prevalence of diabetes needs better strategies for managing and healing diabetic wounds, which frequently present significant hurdles due to complex underlying pathophysiological causes.

The use of artificial intelligence into wound management is expected to revolutionize the assessment and treatment of diabetic wounds. Healthcare workers can give more timely and personalized interventions by leveraging AI's capabilities for accurate wound assessment, remote observation, and predictive analytics. This forward-thinking strategy has the potential to significantly enhance patient outcomes while reducing the pressure on healthcare institutions.

Ayan Mondal[1], Atul Kabra*[1]

Furthermore, personalized medicine offers a promising opportunity to modify treatments based on specific patient features such as genetic makeup and comorbidities. Healthcare practitioners can improve treatment effectiveness and lessen adverse effects by personalizing therapies to each patient's specific needs. This patient-centered paradigm tackles not only the biological variables that influence wound healing, but also the lifestyle and nutritional factors that are critical for recovery. Research into novel medicines such as gene therapy, nanotechnology, and bioengineered grafts is opening the road for ground-breaking treatments that could improve tissue regeneration and repair. These cutting-edge therapies have the potential to provide solutions for individuals suffering from chronic and non-healing wounds, improving their overall quality of life.

www.ingramcontent.com/pod-product-compliance
Lightning Source LLC
Chambersburg PA
CBHW070140230526
45472CB00004B/1618